RESPIRATORY SYNCYTIAL VIRUS

INTO THE HEALING PROCESSES OF
RESPIRATORY SYNCYTIAL VIRUS

DR. J. WALLER

Contents

INTRODUCTION

Respiratory Syncytial Virus, or RSV for short, is a common respiratory virus that can afflict individuals of all ages. It is especially well-known for its ability to induce respiratory tract and lung infections. RSV can affect adults, particularly the elderly or those with compromised immune systems, but it is primarily responsible for respiratory illnesses in young children.

RSV can cause anything from minor cold-like symptoms, including a runny nose and cough, to more serious conditions, like pneumonia or bronchiolitis. When an infected individual coughs or sneezes, the virus spreads by respiratory droplets and can remain on surfaces for several hours.

Preventive measures are essential, particularly for young children, and consistent hand washing is one way to lower the risk of RSV transmission. Hospitalization might be required in extreme circumstances, especially for young children or those with underlying medical issues.

Given the widespread impact of RSV, researchers and medical professionals are always working to discover vaccinations and therapies for the virus.

CHAPTER ONE

Transfer and Propagation

Respiratory droplets, which are microscopic liquid particles discharged into the air when an infected person talks, coughs, or sneezes, are the main way that RSV spreads. Those who are close to the sick person can then inhale these droplets, which is how the virus is spread.

RSV can also linger on surfaces for several hours, and an individual might become infected by touching their face especially their mouth or nose after coming into contact with an infected surface or object.

The virus is extremely contagious, particularly in crowded settings like hospitals and daycare facilities. To reduce the danger of transmission during RSV epidemics, it's critical to practice proper hygiene, such as frequent handwashing.

Fall and winter are the seasons when RSV is most prevalent, and outbreaks frequently take place in neighborhoods, daycare centers, and medical facilities. Because older adults, infants, and young children are especially susceptible to serious problems from RSV, it is imperative to take preventive steps, such as concealing coughs and sneezes and avoiding close contact with ill people.

Symptoms and Indications

Respiratory Syncytial Virus (RSV) symptoms can range in intensity and mimic the symptoms of the flu or common cold. The following are some typical indications and symptoms of RSV:

Coughing: RSV is frequently accompanied by persistent coughing. A minor cough may begin and develop into a more severe and ongoing one.

Runny Nose: Runny or stuffy noses are frequently the result of RSV infections causing nasal congestion.

Fever: A fever can range in severity and is a common symptom. It could be modest in certain situations and higher in others.

Sneezing: RSV can induce sneezing, similar to many other respiratory infections, which helps the virus spread.

Wheezing: RSV can occasionally cause wheezing and breathing difficulties, particularly in young children. This is more frequent in more serious situations and could mean that the lower respiratory tract is involved.

Breathing Problems: Breathing problems, including rapid breathing, are common in infants and early children and may indicate a more serious infection.

Reduced Appetite: Young children and infants may exhibit a diminished desire to eat, which can result in dehydration.

While RSV infections are typically mild and self-limiting, it's crucial to remember that they can be more severe in some populations, including newborns, the elderly, and people with compromised immune systems. Severe instances may require medical treatment and occasionally hospitalization due to the possibility of pneumonia or bronchiolitis. It's best to get medical help right away if you think you may have RSV, especially in groups that are susceptible.

Diagnosis and Assessment

Respiratory Syncytial Virus (RSV) diagnosis usually entails a mix of laboratory tests and clinical examination. The following is how medical practitioners might handle the diagnosis:

Clinical Assessment:

Medical History: The physician will inquire about the patient's symptoms, including their onset, intensity, and course.

Physical Examination: To evaluate respiratory symptoms such coughing, wheezing, and trouble breathing, a comprehensive physical examination may be carried out.

Laboratory Examinations:

Nasal or Throat Swab: To check for the presence of RSV, a swab sample from the nose or throat may be obtained. Polymerase chain reaction (PCR) testing or fast antigen testing are frequently used for this.

Blood Tests: To determine whether RSV antibodies are present, a blood sample may occasionally be obtained.

Imaging Research:

Chest X-ray: To look for evidence of pneumonia or bronchiolitis, a chest X-ray may be taken if there are significant respiratory symptoms.

Additional Examinations:

Monitoring Oxygen Saturation: When respiratory distress occurs, keeping an eye on oxygen saturation levels can assist determine how serious the infection is.

It is significant to remember that the choice to conduct diagnostic tests may be influenced by the patient's age, the severity of their symptoms, and the existence of underlying medical disorders. Clinical signs are frequently used to detect RSV infections, and laboratory testing is not usually required, particularly in mild cases.

It's critical to get medical help right away if you think you may have RSV or if your symptoms are severe. Early detection and treatment are crucial, especially for vulnerable groups including elderly people and newborns.

Preventive Techniques

Using a variety of tactics is necessary to stop the spread of the Respiratory Syncytial Virus (RSV), particularly in environments where the virus is more likely to proliferate. Here are a few crucial preventative steps:

Hand Sanitization:

One of the best strategies to stop the transmission of RSV is to wash your hands often with soap and water.

If soap and water are not available, use hand sanitizers with alcohol base.

Steer clear of close contact:

Refrain from intimate contact with sick people, especially if they exhibit respiratory infection symptoms.

Pneumonia Etiquette:

When you sneeze or cough, cover your mouth and nose with your elbow or a tissue.

Throw away tissues correctly, and then wash your hands right away.

Empty and Rinse:

Doorknobs, toys, and worktops are examples of surfaces that should be cleaned and disinfected on a regular basis.

Since RSV can live on surfaces for several hours, transmission risk can be decreased by routine cleaning.

Separate Ill Persons:

To stop the illness from spreading to others, make every effort to keep the afflicted member of your family as isolated as possible.

Refrain from sharing towels and other personal items.

Immunization (if accessible):

While there isn't a particular RSV vaccine for every age group, some populations—like premature babies or those with specific medical conditions may be given a prophylactic drug called palivizumab during RSV season.

Encourage the health of your respiratory system:

Promote healthy breathing practices, such as abstaining from smoking inside since smoke irritates the respiratory system.

CHAPTER TWO

Educate Healthcare Professionals and Caregivers:

Educate parents, caregivers, and medical professionals on RSV symptoms, preventative measures, and when to seek medical assistance.

It's vital to remember that RSV is extremely contagious, and that prevention is especially important in places like childcare centers and hospitals where vulnerable populations are present. Although total prevention of RSV is not possible, these precautions can greatly lower the chance of transmission.

Since there is no particular antiviral medicine for treating RSV infections, supportive care is the mainstay of treatment for respiratory syncytial virus (RSV). The following are some typical methods for handling RSV:

Symptomatic Management:

Fever and congestion of the nose can be treated with over-the-counter drugs. These, however, are to be used cautiously on small children and under a doctor's supervision.

Fluid Consumption:

Making sure you're getting enough fluids is important, especially for babies and young kids whose lower appetite puts them at risk of dehydration.

Treatment using Oxygen:

To maintain appropriate blood oxygen levels in extreme cases, oxygen therapy may be required, especially in babies.

Bedding in:

Severe RSV infections may need to be hospitalized for intensive observation and supportive care, particularly in young children or those with underlying medical issues.

Bronchodilators:

Bronchodilators are sometimes used to treat wheeze and facilitate breathing. Healthcare professionals continue to disagree on their efficacy in RSV patients, nevertheless.

In the event of a subsequent bacterial infection, antibiotics:

Antibiotics are ineffective against viruses such as RSV; nevertheless, they might be administered in the event that a subsequent bacterial infection is identified or suspected.

It's crucial to remember that antiviral drugs, similar to those used to treat influenza, are not usually recommended for RSV. Early intervention and prevention are crucial, particularly for vulnerable groups. A monoclonal antibody called palivizumab is available for those infants at high risk in order to avoid severe

RSV infection; however, it is not a treatment for infections that are currently active.

If you think you may have an RSV infection, you should always see a doctor, especially if it affects young children, the elderly, or someone with underlying medical issues. The severity of symptoms and consequences can be lessened with early detection and effective treatment.

Populations at High Risk

There are certain groups of people who are thought to be more vulnerable to serious consequences from respiratory syncytial virus (RSV) infections. Among these at-risk demographics are:

Young Children and Infants:

Babies' immature immune and respiratory systems put them at risk for severe RSV infections, especially if they are born before 29 weeks of pregnancy.

Senior Citizens:

Due to the weakened immune system associated with aging, older adults especially those 65 years of age and above may be more susceptible to severe RSV infections.

People with Deflated Immune Systems:

Severe RSV infections are more common in people with compromised immune systems, whether as a result of immunosuppressive drugs or illnesses like HIV/AIDS.

People with Long-Term Medical Conditions:

More severe RSV infections can occur in people with heart disorders, chronic lung diseases (such as chronic obstructive pulmonary disease, or COPD), and certain other chronic medical conditions.

People Affected by Neuromuscular Disorders:

Due to respiratory muscle weakness, those with neuromuscular abnormalities, such as muscular dystrophy, may be more susceptible to complications from RSV.

People residing in extended-care facilities:

Due to shared facilities and close quarters, residents of nursing homes and long-term care facilities are more vulnerable.

Those who look after high-risk individuals:

Family members and caregivers of high-risk persons, especially young children, should exercise caution since they may spread the virus to other individuals who are more vulnerable.

During the RSV season, high-risk newborns may benefit from preventive interventions such the monoclonal antibody palivizumab to lower their chance of developing a serious infection. People who are in high-risk categories should generally take particular care, maintain proper cleanliness, and get medical help as soon as they notice any symptoms of a respiratory infection.

Although the majority of Respiratory Syncytial Virus (RSV) episodes are moderate and self-limiting, serious infections, particularly in specific populations, might result in problems. The following are a few possible long-term consequences and problems of RSV:

Bronchiolitis:

Bronchiolitis, or inflammation of the tiny airways in the lungs, is frequently caused by RSV. Breathing difficulties, wheezing, and coughing may follow from this.

Pneumonia:

Pneumonia, an illness that inflames the lungs' air sacs, can result from severe RSV infections. More severe respiratory symptoms may arise from this.

Infections of the ears:

RSV, especially in young infants, can lead to the development of ear infections.

Intolerance of Asthma:

According to certain research, there may be a connection between early RSV infection and a later-life higher risk of developing asthma or exacerbating pre-existing asthma.

Chronic Respiratory Problems:

Severe RSV infections can occasionally result in long-term respiratory problems and a higher risk of respiratory infections, particularly in newborns and early children.

Bedding in:

Severe RSV infections may necessitate hospitalization for supportive care and monitoring, particularly in high-risk groups such as the elderly and babies.

It's crucial to remember that most people recover completely from RSV with no lasting effects. But individuals who are more likely to experience serious consequences might require more extensive medical attention.

Mitigating the risk of problems linked to RSV requires implementation of preventive measures, timely identification of symptoms, and rapid medical intervention. Furthermore, research is still being conducted to identify treatment and preventative techniques for RSV infections as well as to comprehend any potential long-term repercussions.

Emotional Health and Coping Mechanisms

It can be difficult to deal with the effects of RSV, particularly when a loved one is impacted. The following coping mechanisms and advice can help you keep your emotional health:

CHAPTER THREE

Remain Up to Date:

Learn about RSV, its symptoms, and the available treatments. Certain anxiety can be reduced by being aware of the condition.

Seek Assistance:

Make connections with loved ones, friends, or support groups that may have gone through comparable experiences. Sharing worries and experiences can help one feel less alone.

Interact with Medical Professionals:

Keep lines of communication open and honest with medical experts. Ask questions, get clarification on treatment plans, and voice any concerns you may have.

Observe Self-Care:

Never forget to put your own health first. Make sure you are receiving adequate sleep, eating a healthy diet, and self-care time. If you are a caregiver, this is really crucial.

Maintain Contact:

Maintain contact with your circle of social support. Keeping in touch with friends and family via phone conversations, video chats, or in-person visits can give emotional support.

Have Reasonable Expectations:

Recognize that RSV recovery could take some time. Be patient with the process and set reasonable expectations for the rate of progress.

Communicate Your Emotions:

It's acceptable to have a wide range of feelings, such as anxiety, concern, and frustration. Seek out constructive outlets for your emotions, such as writing in a journal, speaking with a friend, or, if necessary, obtaining professional counseling.

Concentrate on the Good:

See the bright side of everything, especially under difficult circumstances. Celebrate little accomplishments and advancements while keeping an optimistic attitude.

Think About Expert Assistance:

If the emotional toll starts to become too much to bear, think about getting professional mental health assistance. They can offer direction and assistance when things get tough.

Keep in mind that coping mechanisms might differ from person to person, so it's critical to determine what is most effective for you and your family. When you need assistance, don't be afraid to ask for it; also, give your physical and mental health first priority.

CONCLUSION

In summary, the common respiratory virus known as Respiratory Syncytial Virus (RSV) can afflict people of all ages, but it especially affects young children, the elderly, and people with compromised immune systems. Serious infections can result in problems including pneumonia and bronchiolitis, even though the majority of cases only cause minor symptoms akin to the common cold.

The management of RSV mostly entails prevention, which involves hand hygiene, avoiding close contact with sick people, and maintaining clean shared surfaces. Serious complications are more likely to occur in high-risk populations, which include elderly people, prematurely born newborns, and people with underlying medical disorders.

The mainstay of treatment for RSV is supportive care, which aims to control symptoms and avoid complications. Severe cases could necessitate hospitalization, particularly in populations that are more susceptible.

Whether you are the patient or the caregiver, learning more about RSV, getting support, and making self-care a priority are all necessary for emotional survival. Even though most RSV patients recover completely, research is still being done to better understand potential long-term impacts and develop prevention measures.

Research, preventive, and healthcare practices will all continue to advance as our knowledge of respiratory viruses grows, helping to better manage and lessen the effects of RSV on public health.

THE END